Frequently Asked Questions

all about
green tea

VICTORIA DOLBY MPH

AVERY PUBLISHING GROUP

Garden City Park • New York

The information contained in this book is based upon the research and personal and professional experiences of the author. They are not intended as a substitute for consulting with your physician or other health care provider. Any attempt to diagnose and treat an illness should be done under the direction of a health care professional.

The publisher does not advocate the use of any particular health care protocol, but believes the information in this book should be available to the public. The publisher and author are not responsible for any adverse effects or consequences resulting from the use of any of the suggestions, preparations, or procedures discussed in this book. Should the reader have any questions concerning the appropriateness of any procedure or preparation mentioned, the author and the publisher strongly suggest consulting a professional health care advisor.

ISBN: 0-89529-890-2

Printed in the United States of America

10   9   8   7   6   5   4   3   2   1

Contents

*To my mother, Jill-anna Dolby Goodness, who first
introduced me to the pleasures of morning tea.*

Introduction

You may enjoy green tea for its light, subtle taste, but did you know you are doing your body a favor every time you drink it? Green tea is far more than just another refreshing beverage. It has long been renowned as an herbal healer.

You may be hearing about green tea for the first time, but the news about green tea isn't new at all in some parts of the world. Green tea has been revered in China and Japan since ancient times as a tonic for keeping the body and soul in top form.

While it is known that tea plants originated in Southeast Asia, the story of tea's beginnings as a social and medicinal beverage is less clear. Tea's earliest days are shrouded in mystery. One often-repeated bit of folklore contends that tea was first introduced by the Chinese emperor Shen Nong. One day, when the emperor was boiling water to drink, as was his habit, a leaf from a nearby bush wafted into his pot. He allowed it to brew in the water, and he drank the resulting liquid. The emperor was pleased with this concoction. Not long after, in 2737 BCE, he noted in a medical book that tea had to ability to quench thirst, fight fatigue, and lift the spirits.

In the more than 4,000 years since then, tea has been credited with many more health benefits. In fact, in the thirteenth century, Eisai Myo-an, the founder of Zen Buddhism in Japan, wrote a small book about tea entitled *Tea Drinking Is Good for Health*. In this book, he wrote that drinking tea conferred many benefits, namely as a cure for lack of appetite and diseases caused by poor-quality drinking water, as well as for paralysis, boils, and beriberi, a B-vitamin deficiency disease.

Modern scientific research has now confirmed many of the traditionally held beliefs about green tea. There is no longer any question that green tea offers an incredible array of life-enhancing and even life-preserving properties—all the while being easy to use and inexpensive. And it also tastes great!

Why not pour a cup of tea to sip while you read on about this amazing beverage. *All About Green Tea* starts out by answering your basic questions about what green tea is and how it differs from other types of tea. The active ingredients in green tea, especially the antioxidant compounds and caffeine, are thoroughly explained. Subsequent chapters detail the benefits that green tea offers with respect to cancer, heart disease, immune function, longevity, mental acuity, diabetes, ulcers, weight control, osteoporosis, and dental health. Finally, there is a chapter explaining how to incorporate green tea into your life, and a glossary that will help you understand new terms.

All About Green Tea is your one-stop shop for all the information you need to bring the benefits of that ancient healer, green tea, into your life.

1.

Understanding Green Tea

If you are like most Americans, when you feel like having a cup of tea, you probably brew up one of the more familiar black teas, like Earl Grey, English breakfast, or any of the popular name-brand blended teas available at your local supermarket. But the world of tea also includes the less well known green tea. Heading off the beaten track and enjoying green tea can have substantial health benefits. In this chapter, you will find out what the differences are between green and black teas. You will learn about the healing secret ingredients in tea—polyphenols— and why green tea, as the richest source of these polyphenols, has so much to offer. Finally, you will find answers to other basic questions about green tea—its caffeine content and the other nutrients it contains.

Q. Why should I be interested in green tea?

A. Chances are you have enjoyed an occasional cup of green tea at an Asian restaurant. What you probably didn't realize is that you were drinking an ancient healing beverage. Green tea has been prized as a healthful tonic for more than 4,000 years.

But historical precedent is not the only thing on green tea's side. Modern research has turned its eye to this beverage and reports that green tea has many real health benefits. Some of this exciting research points to a link between green tea and cancer prevention. And that's not all. Other research shows that tea, and green tea in particular, helps to bolster the heart's resistance to cardiovascular diseases, increase longevity, detoxify the body, boost immune function, and even prevent cavities.

Q. What makes green tea different from black tea?

A. Although green and black teas start out as leaves from the same plant—*Camellia sinensis*, a shrubby tree native to Southeast Asia—different processing methods lead to very different end products. In their natural state, tea leaves contain enzymes that cause the leaves to become oxidized after picking. When making green tea, processors lightly steam or gently heat the leaves to stop the oxidation process. This processing is so minimal that green tea can be consumed the same day the leaves are picked. On the other hand, tea leaves destined to become black tea are allowed to oxidize and undergo considerably more processing, including a fermentation process that produces the dark-brown and even reddish color of black tea.

Unfortunately, the very process that leads to black tea's distinctive look and taste destroys compounds called polyphenols that are present in the freshly plucked leaves. It is the polyphenols that are associated with the long list of health benefits of green tea. Thus, despite its stronger color and flavor, black tea is a pale shadow of its green cousin as far as health benefits are concerned. Because it is processed as little as possible, green tea retains its original polyphenols. Of all the types of tea available today, green tea has the highest levels of polyphenols.

Q. Does this mean I shouldn't drink black tea?

A. Not at all. Although green tea is superior, black tea is not without health value. And because so many more people currently drink black tea than green tea (the black varieties account for approximately 80 percent of the tea drunk worldwide), this beverage provides a certain level of health benefits if only due to the volume consumed. Studies that track disease rates in countries where people primarily drink black tea indicate that there is indeed some degree of disease protection from drinking black tea. Of course, the health protection would probably be even greater if these people were brewing green tea in their teapots, since green tea provides far greater levels of the beneficial polyphenols.

Q. What are polyphenols, anyway, and what exactly do they do?

A. Polyphenols are a group of naturally occuring phytochemicals (plant chemicals). The polyphenols in tea—which, by the way, account for the pungency and unique flavor of tea—have amazing antioxidant potential. Antioxidants, as you probably know, are substances that protect the body from free radicals. Free radicals are highly reactive molecules and fragments of molecules that can damage the body at the cellular level, helping to set the stage for cancer, heart disease, and many other degenerative diseases. Antioxidants deactivate free radicals, minimizing this damage and protecting the body from disease.

There are many types of antioxidants, including vitamins, minerals, enzymes, and other substances. Polyphenols—which are found in tea as well as in apples, grapes, onions, and many other plants—are a fairly large class of antioxidants. Researchers working with tea have been impressed with green tea's antioxidant potential. Some experts have said that the antioxidant activity of polyphenols seems to be superior to that of the better known antioxidants vitamin C and vitamin E.

There are four primary polyphenols in green tea: epicatechin, epicatechin gallate, epigallocatechin, and epigallocatechin gallate. Sometimes these polyphenols are collectively referred to as *catechins*. You don't have to bother learning to pronounce their names, but you should know that epigallocatechin gallate (EGCG for short) stands out as a powerful antioxidant and health-booster.

Q. Do the other types of tea also contain these beneficial polyphenols?

A. As mentioned earlier, the amount of processing that tea leaves undergo determines how much of the original polyphenols will be retained in the final product. Green tea, with the least processing, retains the most polyphenols—and therefore the most antioxidant potential. Black tea has less.

There is one other type of tea that falls somewhere in between green and black teas. This is oolong tea. Oolong tea is partially fermented, which means that it has a slightly stronger taste than green tea, yet is more delicate than the fully fermented black tea. This partial fermentation process also means that oolong tea contains lower levels of polyphenols than green tea but higher levels than black tea. Oolong tea is the least well known type of tea, accounting for only one percent of yearly tea consumption.

Chi-Tang Ho, PhD, and colleagues from the Department of Food Science and the Center for Advanced Food Technology at Rutgers University recently compared the free-radical-fighting ability of twelve different types of tea, including several varieties of green, oolong, and black teas. Not surprisingly, Ho found that green tea had the highest yields of polyphenols, particularly EGCG. As expected, oolong tea was in the middle, and black tea (as a result of its fermentation process) had the lowest polyphenol yield.

Studies of tea drinkers support the laboratory evidence that shows green tea to be a more effective scavenger of free radicals. One study assigned one group of five adults to drink about two cups of green tea daily, while another group of five adults drank the same amount of black tea. The antioxidant capability of their blood was measured before they drank the tea and at thirty, fifty, and eighty minutes thereafter. Both the green and the black teas improved the antioxidant capability of the blood. However, green tea was six times more powerful than black tea in this regard. The increase in antioxidant function peaked within thirty minutes for the green-tea drinkers and within fifty minutes for those drinking black tea. So although both types of tea act as antioxidants, green tea acts more quickly and more strongly.

Q. Does green tea contain caffeine?

A. Like most other popular hot beverages, green tea does contain caffeine. And the caffeine found in tea is the basis for its reputation as an uplifting beverage, since caffeine is a central nervous system stimulant. If you are like most Americans, you probably consume some caffeine each day—most likely in coffee or soft drinks. You may even be in the select group (about one-third of Americans) who regularly drink tea for your caffeine "fix."

How you prepare your tea affects its caffeine content. Brewing a cup of tea results in 20 to 90 mg of caffeine. Instant or iced teas have about half this amount. Caffeine levels also vary between types of tea. Black teas contain the greatest amounts of caffeine. Oolong teas have about half as much, and green teas have only about one-third the caffeine of black teas. For the sake of comparison, the average cup of coffee provides 60 to 160 mg of caffeine; a can of cola provides approximately 50 mg of caffeine; and a one-ounce chocolate bar provides 1 to 15 mg of caffeine.

Q. What effect does the caffeine in green tea have in the body?

A. Although the pick-me-up effect of tea isn't as strong as that of a cup of coffee, you may have noticed that the caffeine in tea does act as a stimulant—for both the body and the brain.

Moderate amounts of caffeine can increase the

body's basal metabolic rate by approximately 10 percent, an effect that lasts about four hours. Your basal metabolic rate is the amount of energy your body requires to maintain the basic functions of breathing, pumping blood, and maintaining body temperature. The higher your basal metabolic rate, the more calories you burn per minute. The thermogenic (fat-burning) effect of caffeine may be helpful if you are trying to lose weight. If your body burns up more calories, it may be easier for you to achieve a negative calorie balance—that is, to burn more calories than you consume—and for weight loss to occur. However, the potential weight-loss benefit from caffeine alone is minimal at best.

Q. Don't some people have adverse reactions to caffeine?

A. Overdoing it with caffeine, no matter what the source, can give you the jitters. Other negative effects that have been attributed to excessive caffeine intake include frequent urination, diarrhea, insomnia, anxiety, heartburn, and irritability. The amount of caffeine that leads to each of these symptoms varies from person to person. Caffeine-related insomnia shows great variation among different individuals. In general, the sleep-delaying effect of consuming caffeine is greatest for people who are not regularly exposed to it. Of course, pregnant women should steer clear of all sources of caffeine, and, if possible, avoid caffeine a few weeks prior to conception.

The most dreaded side effect from caffeine is caffeine withdrawal syndrome. In this condition, which affects people who habitually consume caffeine over a period of time, symptoms of nervousness, headache, nausea, and muscle tension develop between twelve and twenty-four hours after the last ingestion of caffeine. These withdrawal symptoms are at their most severe during the second day of caffeine withdrawal and can continue for up to a week.

Q. What other substances does tea contain?

A. Tea contains very small amounts of a wide range of nutrients. Vitamin C tops the list. But, as with the polyphenols, vitamin C levels are higher (ten times higher) in green tea than in black tea. Other vitamins found in varying amounts in tea are vitamin B_2 (riboflavin), vitamin D, vitamin K, and the carotenoids (beta-carotene and related compounds).

Tea also contains small amounts of a wide variety of minerals, notably manganese and selenium. Tea, and green tea in particular, is also a source of fluoride—the mineral well known for fighting cavities. Research into the dental benefits of green tea confirms that green tea does, in fact, reduce the incidence of dental cavities. This may, in part, be due to the fluoride content of tea.

Q. All of this sounds great. But are there any downsides to drinking green tea?

A. Not that we know of. Several years ago, concerns were raised that drinking tea might interfere with the body's absorption and use of iron, which in turn could increase the risk of anemia. Fortunately, further research has determined that tea does not increase the risk of iron-deficient anemia. Nevertheless, to be prudent, some physicians still recommend that people taking iron supplements should not swallow their pills with tea.

Another concern that was raised was the seemingly high level of the mineral aluminum sometimes found in tea—particularly since an excessive intake of aluminum may be associated with serious bone and brain disorders. Again, further research has taken tea off the hook. The aluminum that is in tea is present in a complex, rather than ionic, form. This means that the type of aluminum in tea is not able to react in the body in harmful ways.

2.

Preventing Cancer

Cancer is a disease in which cells begin to reproduce in an uncontrolled fashion, resulting in tumors that can threaten the functioning of one or more parts of the body. It is one of the most dreaded diseases of the modern world, and for good reason: Worldwide, it claims over 6 million lives each year. Every single day in the United States, more than 1,500 lives are lost to cancer, while another 3,700 people learn that they have this disease.

One of the most puzzling questions confronting modern science is, Why do some people develop cancer, but others don't? The answers appear to lie in differences in genetics, environment, immune function, lifestyle, and diet. Including "anti-cancer" foods in your diet shows tremendous promise as one of the factors that can help tip the scales in your favor. Green tea is among the most promising of these cancer-fighting dietary factors, as we will see in this chapter.

Q. Can something as simple as green tea really help prevent cancer?

A. The reputation of green tea as a health-enhancing beverage can be traced back thousands of years. In the past, many Western scientists dismissed this as folklore. This dismissal changed to respect when epidemiologists (scientists who study the risks of various diseases and numbers of death from those diseases among groups of people) took a closer look at the statistics. They discovered that Asians have a lower risk of getting, or dying from, many diseases that plague most Western countries, including cancer. Even when factors that could affect health— such as access to medical care, smoking, genetic differences, and exposure to pollution—are accounted for, Asians continue to be at the top in worldwide comparisons of disease and health. It seems likely that dietary factors contribute to this discrepancy, and the consumption of green tea ranks high as one of these factors.

Of course, even within Asian countries, disease rates vary from region to region. Take, for example, the Shizuoka Prefecture of Japan, a coastal region southwest of Tokyo. Epidemiologists noticed that this area of Japan had a much lower death rate from cancer for both men and women, compared to that in in the country as a whole. Intrigued by this phenomenon, they decided to delve deeper. They discovered that green tea was a staple beverage in the tea-growing Shizuoka region; people living in this area drank more cups of green tea than average Japanese citizens. It seemed logical, these scientists suggested, that the green-tea drinking of these people contributed to their surprisingly lower cancer rates.

Q. But is that really conclusive evidence for green tea as a cancer-preventer?

A. It's true, the statistical connection between one area of Japan where people citizens drink exceptionally large amounts of green tea and also have lower cancer rates is not enough in and of itself to prove that green tea prevents cancer. But scientists have followed up on this connection with dozens of experiments to determine if their theory is correct. Does green tea really reduce the risk of cancer? Let's see what they found out.

Of the many scientific studies conducted in laboratory petri dishes, animal populations, and even human subjects, one of the most convincing studies was undertaken not in a far-away Asian country, but right here in the United States, in Iowa. Researchers sent a questionnaire to 35,369 middle-aged Iowan women asking questions about their health, lifestyle, and diet, including questions about how much tea they drank on an average day. The epidemiologists then kept an eye on these women for the next eight years, tracking how many developed cancer.

Overall, about 40 percent of these Iowan women drank tea of any variety (green, black, or oolong) at least once a week. Almost 20 percent drank tea every day, and half of this group reported drinking two or more cups daily. The women who drank the most tea were found to have a 10 percent lower incidence of cancer. And when the cancers were broken down by different types, it was found that the frequent tea-drinkers had almost 70 percent fewer cancers of the digestive tract and 40 percent fewer urinary tract cancer cases compared to women who rarely or never drank tea. Clearly, tea is in some way associated with a lower risk of cancer.

Q. If green tea really does reduce the risk of cancer, how does it do it?

A. Once again, the answer goes back to free radicals and the antioxidant potential of green tea (see page 12). Of the various types of cellular damage that can be caused by free radicals, the damage to

DNA (the cells' genetic material) can be the most dangerous. If a cell's DNA is damaged by free radicals, every time the cell reproduces itself it also reproduces the free-radical damage. In fact, the damage can be magnified in the succeeding cellular generations.

The path from damaged DNA to cancer is believed to require an accumulation, over time, of specific DNA defects in specific target cells. The initial free-radical "hit" may occur many years before the cell's transformation to a cancerous state is complete and actual disease is discernible.

According to some free-radical experts, each molecule of DNA in our bodies can (and does) receive thousands of free radical "hits" each day and continue unaffected by the insult. This is because the body is continually replacing and repairing itself in a very efficient manner. But the body is not invincible. If free-radical-damaged DNA is not repaired before a cell divides, the damage becomes permanent, and potentially cancerous. Remember, it is antioxidants that protect cells against free-radical damage. If the levels of antioxidants in your body are low, a particular free-radical hit may fail to be corrected.

This is where green tea comes in. The polyphenols in green tea increase the level of antioxidant in the body—antioxidants that neutralize free radicals before they have a chance to damage the cells' DNA.

Q. So is preventing cancer just a matter of protecting the body from free radicals?

A. That's one important consideration. But free-radical deactivation is not the only way green tea is thought to thwart cancer. Dr. Theresa J. Smith, a researcher at Rutgers University in New Jersey, has been cataloging additional ways that green tea undermines cancer. According to Dr. Smith, green tea prevents strands of DNA from breaking, inhibits uncontrolled cell reproduction, decreases the contact of carcinogens (cancer-causing substances) with cells, blocks the transformation of normal cells into cancer cells, and also slows the progression of cancer.

Another promising way in which green tea prevents cancer is by inhibiting the activation of carcinogens. A study published in the professional journal *Food & Chemical Toxicology* found that rats that were given the equivalent of a human dose of green tea had a lower risk of cancer because "the anticarcinogenic effect of green tea facilitated the metabolism of chemical carcinogens into inactive, readily excretable products." In other words, the green tea kicked potential cancer-causing substances out of the body before they could do any damage.

Although carcinogens are potentially dangerous by themselves, when they are activated by enzymes in the body, they can become particularly nasty. Certain enzymes found in the liver, known as *cytochrome P450 enzymes*, can activate carcinogens. Once activated, the carcinogens can attack DNA and other components of the body's cells. Fortunately, there are many anti-cancer compounds that block the activation of carcinogens by P450 enzymes. Not surprisingly, green tea is among these, and EGCG is the most powerful of the polyphenols with this ability.

Perhaps the researchers at the National Cancer Center Research Institute in Tokyo, Japan, provide the best overall summary of the cancer-preventing abilities of green tea. "We suggest [that] drinking green tea may be one of the most practical methods of cancer prevention available at the present."

Q. Does green tea work to prevent all kinds of cancer, or does it work differently for different cancers?

A. Although green tea has been shown to reduce the overall risk of cancer, the majority of studies have examined green tea (and extracts of green tea) as they relate to cancers that develop in specific organs or tissues of the body. For example, research done in the laboratory and with animal models suggests that green tea extract, either taken orally or applied directly to the skin, offers significant protection against the development of skin cancer caused by exposure to the sun's ultraviolet (UV) rays or cancer-causing chemicals. Santosh K. Katiyar, PhD, of the Department of Dermatology at the Case Western Reserve University in Cleveland, Ohio, is probably the preeminent researcher in the field of skin-cancer prevention. He has conducted several studies investigating green tea's ability to prevent skin cancer in mice. Although future research in people will be needed to confirm his work, things do look promising.

Dr. Katiyar's research found that green tea protects against cancers caused by UV radiation, and that a green-tea cream applied prior to exposure to a carcinogen is highly effective in protecting the skin against cancerous changes. Additional research has found that the progression of skin cancer is also lessened by applying green tea topically. Thus, while green-tea extract shows the most protective effect when it is administered before cancer develops, it is beneficial throughout all stages of the disease. We probably don't have long to wait before green-tea extract is a standard ingredient in sunscreens and skin creams.

Q. Since green tea ends up in the stomach, does it protect against cancer there?

A. Remember the Japanese region of Shizuoka—noted for an unexpectedly low overall cancer incidence? Well, people living in this area have an especially low incidence of stomach cancer. Since the population of this region is known to drink more than average amount of green tea (even by Japanese standards), this relationship sparked several research studies in the area of green tea and stomach cancer. A Japanese study of 139 patients diagnosed with stomach cancer and 2,852 people without cancer found that individuals who drank large quantities of green tea (ten or more cups daily) were much less likely to have cancer of the stomach.

Another study—this one in China and involving 1,422 individuals—found that green-tea drinkers had a 29 percent lower risk for developing cancer of the stomach than those who didn't drink green tea.

Q. Following the path of green tea even further, does it affect the risk of bladder cancer?

A. On its way out of the body, green tea does appear to protect the bladder from cancer. This protection has been studied in groups considered to be at high risk for bladder cancer, namely cigarette smokers and certain industrial workers (including people who worked in the dye, chemical, leather, and rubber industries).

The International Agency for Research on Cancer determined that smokers with a high intake of polyphenols "are partially protected against the harmful effects by tobacco carcinogens within their bladder mucosal cells." Another study, involving 293 bladder-cancer patients and 589 healthy control subjects, found that drinking green tea was correlated with a significantly lower risk of bladder cancer.

Q. What's the story for breast cancer?

A. A link between green tea and a lower risk of breast cancer was suggested after epidemiologists noticed that Japanese women who move to the United States and adopt an American diet quickly assume the breast-cancer risks of American women, while those who continue to live in Japan have a very low risk of breast cancer. It seems to follow that American women could lower their chances of joining the ranks of breast-cancer statistics by emulating a Japanese diet and including green tea in their lives.

Laboratory studies on the green tea-breast cancer connection suggest that green-tea extracts, and EGCG in particular, stop the growth of breast-cancer cells. They do this by interacting with tumor-promoters, hormones, and growth factors to "seal off" the cancer cells. EGCG also fights breast cancer by slowing the growth of breast-cancer cells that tend to grow abnormally fast, which contributes to the spread of the disease.

When researchers at the Nagoya City University Medical School in Nagoya, Japan, tested a series of naturally occurring antioxidants, they discovered that green-tea polyphenols came out on top in terms of preventing breast cancer. Groups of rats were exposed to carcinogens that greatly increase the risk of breast cancer. Some groups were fed a regular diet, while other groups' diets also received different antioxidants. All of the antioxidants improved the survival rates of these animals through the thirty-six weeks of the study. In the rats that developed breast tumors, the number of tumors per rat was lower and the size of the tumors was much smaller in the green-tea group. The researchers conclude that "of the four antioxidants tested, the effects of [green-tea polyphenols] appeared most beneficial since no animals died of mammary tumor during the experiment. One interpretation is that [the polyphenol] GTC inhibited the growth of the mammary tumors."

Q. How about prostate cancer? Does green tea offer any protection?

A. Cancer of the prostate is the most common cancer, and the second most common cause of cancer-related death, in American men. Preliminary research suggests that green tea holds some promise for this type of cancer, although it is far from a first line of defense. Nevertheless, investigators from the Cancer Research Center at the University of Chicago discovered that EGCG from green tea inhibited the growth of prostate tumors and also reduced the size of existing tumors. "It is possible," researchers concluded, "that there is a relationship between the high consumption of green tea and the low incidence of prostate . . . cancers in some Asian countries."

Q. What about smokers? Can they gain any benefits from green tea?

A. Lung cancer is the number one cancer killer of both men and women, and as everyone knows, many cases of lung cancer can be traced to cigarette smoking. Green-tea extract shows promise in guarding against lung cancer. Researchers at the Department of Veterans Affairs Medical Center in Cleveland, Ohio, report that polyphenols extracted from green tea result in 55 percent fewer lung tumors in mice exposed to carcinogens. Japanese researchers discovered that mice given a green-tea infusion to drink had significantly reduced metastasis (spreading) of lung tumors. Other research shows that green tea slashes the number of cancerous and precancerous lesions in mice from 80 percent to 14 percent.

Of the numerous carcinogens in cigarette smoke, one in particular is highly correlated to the development of lung cancer. This is a compund classed as nitrosamine and called NNK. Researchers believe that NNK is activated by the cytochrome P450 enzymes in the liver (see page 27) to become an active carcinogen.

Certain dietary or lifestyle factors must influence the activation of tobacco carcinogens, because even though Japanese men are twice as likely as American men to smoke, the lung cancer mortality rates in Japan are lower than in the United States.

Animal research indicates that the polyphenols in green tea can reverse some of the damage caused by NNK. When mice are treated with NNK, they develop an average of 22.5 lung tumors per mouse. However, when EGCG is added to their drinking water, only 16.1 tumors develop. Based on the amounts of EGCG given to these animals, it would appear that small amounts of EGCG—as little as is found in a daily cup of green tea—would lessen the impact of NNK in human smokers.

Research in human populations supports the results from animal studies. The blood of fifty-two healthy men between the ages of twenty and fifty-two was analyzed for blood markers signaling the presence of tobacco-related carcinogens. The men who regularly drank green tea had the blood profiles of nonsmokers, while those who did not drink green tea showed unhealthy blood levels of tobacco-derived carcinogens. Although the obvious first choice for health is not to smoke, if you do smoke, you may obtain some protection from the carcinogens in tobacco smoke by consuming green tea regularly.

3.

Brimming With Heart Benefits

Cardiovascular diseases take the lives of almost one million Americans each year, more than any other single group of diseases. But there is good news: Green tea can play a role in turning the tide. In this chapter, you will learn about the beneficial effects of green tea on cholesterol, the heart, and blood vessels. You will be especially interested in this chapter if you are concerned about high blood pressure or stroke. Pay particular attention if you are a smoker.

Q. What effect does green tea have on cholesterol?

A. The regular consumption of green tea can be a helpful component of a cholesterol-management

plan. People who drink green tea regularly generally have healthier cholesterol levels than those who
don't. A study in which 1,371 Japanese men over the
age of 40 were interviewed about their diets and
lifestyles found that the consumption of green tea
turned out to be a strong predictor of lower cholesterol levels. The men who drank ten or more cups of
green tea daily had significantly lower cholesterol
levels than those who did not. They also had healthier cholesterol profiles—that is, their levels of low-
density lipoproteins (LDL, the so-called "bad" cholesterol) were lower and their levels of high-density
lipoproteins (HDL, or "good" cholesterol) were
higher in the most dedicated green-tea imbibers.

Similar good news about green tea and cholesterol emerged from a study of 1,306 retiring
Japanese government officials. The men who regularly drank nine or more cups of green tea daily had
total blood-cholesterol levels that were an average
of 8 milligrams per deciliter (mg/dl) lower than
those of the men who drank two cups or less daily.
Now, every 1 percent decrease in your cholesterol
level translates into a 2 percent-lower risk of heart
disease. So if your cholesterol count is 200 mg/dl
(the level considered the upper limit for good
health) and you lower it by 8 mg/dl, you have low-
ered your cholesterol level by 4 percent—which
means, in turn, that you have reduced your risk of

heart disease by 8 percent. This implies that drinking green tea regularly offers a modest, but significant and encouraging, degree of protection against heart disease.

An even larger study—involving more than 20,000 middle-aged Norwegian men and women—reported that cholesterol levels decrease as tea consumption increases. Men drinking five or more cups of tea daily had total cholesterol levels that were an average of 9.3 mg/dl lower than those who drank a cup or less daily. For women, the corresponding figure was 5.8 mg/dl. Furthermore, the study found that those who didn't drink tea were more likely to die from heart attacks than the tea drinkers were. The results of this study are all the more impressive when you consider that Norwegians tend to drink black tea, which contains much lower levels of polyphenols than green tea.

Q. But *how* does green tea protect against heart disease?

A. Once the evidence linking green tea to lower cholesterol levels started to roll in, scientists naturally began to question how green tea might achieve this effect. They found out plenty. For starters, green tea blocks the body's absorption of dietary cholesterol. Quite simply, if your body cannot absorb the cholesterol in the foods you eat, it cannot increase your blood-cholesterol level.

To further clarify this protective effect of green tea, researchers from the Laboratory of Nutrition Chemistry at the Kyushu University School of Agriculture in Japan set up a series of animal experiments. Groups of rats were fed diets rich in cholesterol and saturated fat, with different groups also receiving various green-tea polyphenols. The absorption of cholesterol was found to be markedly inhibited by the polyphenols, and the most effective cholesterol-inhibitor was EGCG (see page 13). Specifically, rats fed a high-cholesterol coconut-oil-based diet absorbed 48.5 percent of the cholesterol in their food, but when EGCG was added to this heart-damaging diet, absorption dropped to a mere 16.7 percent.

The antioxidant capability of green tea cannot be discounted as another way green tea protects the cardiovascular system. When LDL cholesterol is damaged by free radicals through a process called oxidation, it becomes especially adept at promoting heart disease. As antioxidants, green tea's polyphenols help prevent this harmful oxidation.

Q. Can green tea also help prevent strokes?

A. Guarding against strokes is yet another area in which green tea holds great promise. Actually, all polyphenols—those found in green tea and those found in other plants—support healthy circulation. Polyphenols are believed to protect against stroke by acting as antioxidants as well as by preventing blood clots.

For instance, when Dutch researchers tracked the incidence of stroke in 552 men aged fifty to sixty-nine over a period of fifteen years, they found that the men who consumed the most polyphenols experienced 73 percent fewer strokes than those who consumed the least of these compounds. In this study, black tea and apples were the main source of dietary polyphenols—and the tea accounted for 70 percent of the polyphenols in the diets of these men. Taking an even closer look at the data, researchers found that the men who drank approximately five cups of tea each day had a 69 percent lower risk of experiencing a stroke compared to men who drank only about two cups or less daily. Apparently, just a few cups of tea each day can go a long way.

Similarly, a Japanese study of 5,910 middle-aged

women found that strokes were least common in women who drank the most green tea. When these women were followed for four years, strokes were found to be twice as likely in the women who drank less than five cups of green tea daily than in the green-tea lovers.

Q. What about blood pressure? Does green tea have any effect on that?

A. Hypertension (high blood pressure) is known to doctors as the "silent killer." It can progress without symptoms and lead or contribute to heart attack, stroke, internal bleeding, and a host of life-threatening conditions. If your blood pressure is consistently higher than 140/90 when you are at rest, you are likely to be diagnosed with high blood pressure. The first number in this reading is the *systolic pressure*. It represents the pressure in the blood vessel at the moment the heart beats and sends blood into the arteries. This is the peak level of pressure. The second number is the *diastolic pressure*, which is the pressure between heartbeats—the lowest level of pressure in the blood vessels.

The Norwegian study mentioned earlier that investigated green tea and cholesterol levels also reported benefits related to blood pressure. Specifically, it found that systolic pressure was lower in the men and women who had a greater average tea intake. Animal studies support this relationship. For instance, one study found that when mice were subjected to stress, their blood pressure rose accordingly. But adding decaffeinated green tea to their water kept rising blood pressures in check, despite the mounting stress levels.

Q. What does green tea do that causes this effect?

A. It relaxes the blood vessels so that blood can flow more easily. Relaxing the blood vessel walls can be helpful in reducing high blood pressure. Researchers who compared dozens of plants and plant extracts for their ability to relax blood vessels found that green tea was among the best for this purpose. Out of the fifty-four vegetables, fruits, nuts, herbs, spices, and teas that were tested, green tea was ranked number five, and produced a 91 percent relaxation of the endothelium (the lining of blood vessels). Black tea, presumably because it has lower polyphenol levels, relaxed blood vessels by only 66 percent.

Q. Do smokers gain any special benefits?

A. If you smoke, you have heard this advice before: The best thing you can do for your health is to quit. But if you cannot or simply do not want to quit, green tea might help lower the risk of heart disease.

Free-radical damage to the blood vessels is an important contributing factor in the initiation of heart disease. How much free-radical damage the vessels have suffered can be measured by assessing the amount of substances called *lipid peroxides* in the blood. Because of the numerous free radicals in tobacco smoke, smokers tend to have much higher lipid-peroxide levels than nonsmokers. This would account, in part, for smokers' increased risk of heart disease. Yet a Japanese researcher found that heavy smokers who were also among the most dedicated green-tea drinkers (consuming more than ten cups daily) had lipid-peroxide profiles similar to those of nonsmokers. We can therefore assume that drinking significant quantities of green tea regularly may, in part, counteract the damage of tobacco use.

4.

Beating Infection

Despite dramatic progress made in antibiotics and other treatment strategies, infectious diseases remain a major threat to human health. We are all exposed to potentially disease-causing organisms on a daily basis. If it were not for the body's immune system, we would suffer bout after bout of infectious illness. Ultimately, life itself would be impossible.

Unfortunately, natural immunity suffers when we are exposed to toxins, pollutants, and stress (both physical and psychological)—all of which are part of everyday life today. In this chapter, we will explore the ways in which green tea can help boost immunity and fight infection.

Q. What exactly does "boosting immunity" mean, and how can green tea help?

A. Your immune-system response is what determines whether you will succumb to the myriad bacteria, viruses, fungi, and other microorganisms you encounter every day, or whether your body's natural defenses will brush them off and maintain good health. The immune system is an intricate network that includes specialized tissues, organs, and cells, and chemicals secreted by those cells, whose missions are to seek out and destroy foreign invaders before they cause illness.

Some of the key actors in the immune defense system are specialized white blood cells called lymphocytes. Some lymphocytes, called B-cells, are released directly into the bloodstream to monitor the blood for dangerous invaders. Once there, they learn to identify and produce antibodies that attack specific germs. Other lymphocytes, called T-cells, mature in the thymus gland, then emerge to attack infectious agents directly.

Based on experiments they conducted on animals, researchers at the Showa University School of Medicine in Tokyo, Japan, concluded that "EGCG showed strong immunoenhancement of B-cells." In other words, the green-tea polyphenol EGCG boosted the activity of the immune system's B-cells. Another polyphenol, ECG, also had some effect. The researchers also noted that green-tea polyphenols boosted the activity of macrophages (white blood cells that surround and literally consume germs), T-cells, and natural killer cells (activated white cells that go on "seek-and-destroy" missions against invasive cells).

Q. What if my immune system doesn't kill all the germs? Can green tea help that, too?

A. It certainly appears that way. Listen to the findings of Dr. J. M. T. Hamilton-Miller of the Department of Medical Microbiology at the Royal Free Hospital School of Medicine in London. Dr. Hamilton-Miller reviewed the antimicrobial properties of tea and found that tea extracts disarm and even kill many species of bacteria, especially the kinds that cause diarrheal-type diseases. In general, the amount of tea extract that exerts these antibacterial effects is equivalent to the amount you would get drinking tea as a beverage. A word of warning, however: This doesn't mean that if you get a bacterial illness, you should forgo regular antibiotic treatment. But green tea can be used together with antibiotics to help you recover.

Green-tea extracts have been specifically tested

in the prevention of several bacterial infections. Although whooping cough is now uncommon in the United States because of vaccination programs, it remains a problem in other parts of the world. Whooping cough—or, as doctors call it, pertussis—is caused by the bacterium *Bordetella pertussis*. Japanese researchers determined that the polyphenol EGCG in green tea and the compound theaflavin in black tea "might act as [preventive] agents against pertussis infection." This is apparently accomplished in several different ways. First, these compounds seem to keep bacteria from adhering to cells in the body and, thus, from infecting them. EGCG and theaflavin also seem to prevent *Bordetella pertussis* from damaging white blood cells, those important components of the immune system whose job is to destroy infecting organisms. This same group of researchers also found that green and black teas can be used preventively against pneumonia infection.

Cholera is an acute infectious disease of the small intestine, caused by the bacterium *Vibrio cholerae*. It causes profuse watery diarrhea, vomiting, muscle cramps, severe dehydration, depletion of electrolytes, and, sometimes, death. Japanese researchers, supported by the Japanese Cholera Panel of the United States-Japan Cooperative Medical Science Program, took a closer look at the bacteria-fighting effects of green-tea extract in an animal model. They reported that "tea [polyphenols] inhibit the activity of cholera toxin, and protect against cholera infection. . . ." Furthermore, they recommended that physicians consider including polyphenols in their treatment of cholera patients to hasten recovery.

Green-tea polyphenols have also been shown, in laboratory and animal experiments as well as in human trials, to inhibit the growth of *Streptococcus mutans*, the bacteria responsible for dental plaque and cavities (more about this in Chapter 6).

Q. Could green tea help me avoid infections like the flu?

A. It certainly might, since the influenza virus also seems to be inactivated by the polyphenols in green tea. Researchers at the National Institute of Health in Tokyo, Japan, discovered that EGCG binds with the flu virus, thereby preventing it from causing infection.

Many people count on a yearly flu shot to protect them against this illness. However, the influenza virus is continually changing. As a result, the vaccine that protected you last year may not be effective this year. A drug called amantadine is sometimes used to treat influenza, however, it produces many side effects and contributes to the development of resistant strains of the flu virus. Further, amantadine levels need to be 50 to 100 times greater than those of tea polyphenols to produce the same level of influenza-virus deactivation. This suggests great promise for polyphenols in preventing the flu. One animal study supported the anti-influenza action of polyphenols. When a group of mice were infected with the flu virus, all died within ten days. However, a second group of mice were given polyphenols right after being exposed to the virus, and all of these mice survived.

Q. What about one of the most serious infections out there today—HIV? Is there any chance that green tea might help?

A. Research is currently underway regarding green tea and the human immunodeficiency virus (HIV), the virus that causes AIDS. AIDS researchers, despite occasional progress and breakthroughs, remain frustrated in their search for a way to prevent infection with HIV.

It should be stressed that green tea is *not* a miracle breakthrough in the treatment of HIV infection. But once again, the polyphenol EGCG has raised some interest here. It has been reported to inhibit an enzyme called reverse transcriptase, which plays an essential role in the reproduction of HIV. This is the same enzyme that other anti-HIV drugs—including the best known, AZT—seek to inhibit. The problem with most agents that inhibit reverse transcriptase, however, is that they can also interfere with the action of other enzymes that are needed for the reproduction of the body's own DNA. This leads to many undesirable side effects. In laboratory studies, the level of EGCG required to stop the virus from reproducing was five times lower than the level that would interfere with the body's own natural cellular reproduction. Further research is needed to determine whether the same results might be obtained in human subjects, but the initial findings, at least, are encouraging.

5.

Living Longer, Enjoying Life

Green tea is not the long-sought-after fountain of youth, but it just might add a few years to your life. More better than that, green tea may help to add life to your years by protecting against diseases that might otherwise degrade your quality of life along the way.

In this chapter, you will learn how green tea can help you look younger and stay smart—while you are living longer. And you will discover how green tea brings added benefits to anyone concerned about diabetes, ulcers, osteoporosis, liver health, or weight management.

Q. Do green-tea drinkers really live longer?

A. Green-tea lovers do appear to live longer. One study that uncovered this fact examined the relationship of green tea to longevity by following the lives of 3,380 Japanese women for nine years. These women were all taught the Japanese tea ceremony in Tokyo, and were age fifty or older. Green tea is an essential component of the Japanese tea ceremony, so the researchers felt it was safe to assume that these women were greater-than-average green-tea drinkers. The death of any woman in this group between 1980 and 1988 was recorded. Comparing the numbers of deaths among women in this group with the mortality rates of other Japanese women, both in Tokyo and in Japan as a whole, during this same time period, researchers found that fewer of the "hard-core" green-tea drinkers died. They concluded that this indicated "the possibility that green tea is a protective factor for several fatal diseases."

Although it is sometimes hard to extrapolate from animal research to effects on humans, work that has been done with animals supports the idea that tea may have life-extending effects. Chinese researchers found that fruit flies, which generally live only fifteen days, stay alive a stunning forty days—more than twice their normal life span—when jasmine tea was added to their drinking water. Japanese researchers at the Nagasaki University School of Medicine found similar results in studies done on laboratory rats. When rats were given tea extract containing the polyphenol EGCG in their water, their life spans were significantly prolonged. The researchers conducting this study attributed green tea's apparent relationship to longevity to its free-radical-fighting abilities.

Q. Can green tea keep me *looking* younger, too?

A. Free radicals can damage the skin's appearance and contribute to an older-looking face. The sun's ultraviolet rays are a primary source of free radicals and a major foe to firm, youthful skin. Frequent or prolonged sun exposure is a major contributor to premature aging and wrinkles. Supplementing your diet with antioxidants, such as the polyphenols found in green tea, defuses free radicals and, therefore, a source of wrinkles.

When free radicals attack collagen, the skin's structural protein, skin loses its elasticity. Antioxidants, including polyphenols, protect the skin from this damage. In addition, green tea's polyphenols are able to reduce the activity of collagenase, the enzyme that breaks down collagen. While green tea can't promise to act as an herbal face-lift, it might help minimize the damage skin experiences in day-to-day life.

Q. Do we really know whether green tea creates healthier people? Couldn't it be that healthier people just happen to be tea drinkers?

A. A debate is brewing between certain researchers as to whether tea drinking itself reduces the risk of disease, or whether tea drinkers tend to have other healthy habits that reduce their risk. In other words, it has been suggested that tea just seems to improve health because tea drinkers happen to be healthier people to start with.

It does appear to be true that tea-drinkers on the whole are healthier than average in terms of diet and lifestyle. For example, people who report drinking significant quantities of tea are less likely than the general population to smoke and more likely to eat a healthy diet and take dietary supplements. But the disease-preventing abilities of green tea should not be discounted. Drinking tea provides health benefits in and of itself.

Q. Can drinking green tea keep my mind in top shape?

A. As they age, most people experience some decline in memory, learning, and concentration. The underlying cause of this decline is partially accounted for by the accumulation of free-radical-damaged brain cells that, over time, manifest themselves as declining mental function. Antioxidants—including the green-tea polyphenol EGCG—are a great way to protect the brain from free-radical attacks. Researchers at the Science University of Tokyo, Japan have said they believe that "the effect of tea catechins in promoting neurons of normal learning ability . . . may be related to their ability to scavenge active oxygen species. [As such, they] . . . might become useful for protecting humans from senile disorders such as dementia." In other words, by protecting the brain cells from free-radical attacks, green-tea polyphenols may help people retain their ability to learn and remember.

The caffeine content of green tea may be another factor in this beverage's support of clear thinking. Scientific studies show that caffeine (from any source) enhances a person's performance on tasks related to perception, learning, and reasoning, particularly in the areas of reaction time, accurate appraisal of spatial relationships, and certain aspects of memory. Caffeine also staves off boredom and mental fatigue. Caffeine has also been linked to increased energy, feelings of well-being, and motivation to work.

Q. You mentioned specific benefits for diabetics. What benefits are those?

A. Diabetes, although found around the globe, is most prevalent in the United States. By some estimates, as many as half of all the world's diabetics live in the United States. Our "affluent" diet and lifestyle are often to blame.

Diabetes is a condition in which the body fails to produce sufficient amounts of insulin, a hormone that permits the cells to use glucose (blood sugar, their primary fuel) to carry on their essential activities. As a result, the level of sugar in the blood rises while the cells are starved for nutrition. Although it is certainly not the first-line treatment for diabetes, green tea may provide some benefits for diabetics. In diabetic animals, green-tea polyphenols have been shown to bring high blood-sugar levels back down to normal. In addition, the insulin-producing cells of these animals, which had been inactive, regenerated and regained their proper function. Other researchers report that polyphenols, besides promoting the secretion of insulin, also have insulin-like action in the body. In all, the animal research suggests that tea may have both a preventive and curative effect on diabetes. There is a word of caution, however: One isolated study suggested that children who regularly consumed tea had an increased risk of developing type I diabetes, also known as insulin-dependent or juvenile-onset diabetes.

Q. You also mentioned ulcers. What is the green-tea connection there?

A. Stomach ulcers are a common problem, affecting one out of every ten Americans at some time in his or her life. Green-tea polyphenols may help prevent ulcers. In one animal study, polyphenols showed an 80 percent success rate in preventing stomach ulcers. Another study reported that giving normally brewed black tea to laboratory rats inhibited the formation of ulcers, even when the rats were given aspirin and other medications that increase the risk of ulcers.

Q. Is there a weight-loss connection to green tea?

A. To start with, a cup of tea (without added sugar or milk) provides only four calories, which certainly makes this beverage acceptable for any weight-loss diet. Further, weight-loss experts theorize that green tea may reduce the rate and amount of carbohydrate absorption, without threatening a person's nutritional status. Green tea causes carbohydrates to be released slowly, preventing sharp spikes in blood-insulin levels and in turn promoting the burning of fat. The "extra," unabsorbed carbohydrates are disposed of in the stool. This also can be beneficial; it bulks up the stools and helps to prevent constipation, a common occurrence in dieters.

Although the body of literature supporting the use of green tea as a diet aid is small, the preliminary studies that do exist are promising. In one study, sixty obese middle-aged women were put on a diet supplying 1,800 calories a day. One group took green-tea supplements with breakfast, lunch, and dinner; another group took placebo ("dummy") pills. After two weeks on this regimen, the women taking green-tea extract lost twice as much weight as those in the placebo group did. The results were even more impressive after a month;

the green-tea users had triple the weight loss, on average, as compared with women who were simply dieting.

Part of the reason green tea promotes weight loss is explained by its caffeine content. Caffeine increases the body's basal metabolic rate (the amount of energy required to maintain the basic functions of breathing, pumping blood, and body temperature). This is referred to as a thermogenic effect, and it may boost weight loss efforts by helping the body burn more calories. The potential effect on weight loss is small, but nevertheless significant.

Pouring a cup of green tea with dinner isn't going to be a miracle weight-loss aid—a healthy diet and regular exercise simply cannot be replaced—but if you develop a fondness for this beverage, it can certainly help.

Q. What about green tea and osteoporosis?

A. The research on green tea and osteoporosis is in its early stages—much more needs to be done. However, we do know that building strong, dense, healthy bones is the best prevention against osteoporosis. This is a continuous process. Bones are constantly remodeling themselves, as old bone is removed and new bone is deposited. If the removal happens more quickly than new deposits, osteoporosis becomes more likely.

According to one animal study, green-tea polyphenols can reduce the excessive reabsorption of old bone that can lead to bone loss. Epidemiological studies support this theory.

Q. How about the liver? Does green tea help this important organ?

A. Promoting a healthy liver is one of the ways that tea's polyphenols support good health. In particular, polyphenols help the liver's enzyme system to function more effectively and protect the liver itself from the toxins it is detoxifying. Additionally, research in animals suggests that green tea can prevent injury to the liver from viral hepatitis. Turning back to people, Japanese epidemiologists surveyed the diets and tracked the liver health of 1,371 adult men and discovered that "increased consumption of green tea, especially more than 10 cups a day, was related to decreased concentrations of hepatological markers" (signs that indicate damage to liver cells).

6.

Promoting Dental Health

I n Japan and China, it is customary to take some green tea after every meal. This habit has long been believed to maintain a healthy mouth. And this traditional preventive medicine is now being proven by modern research to have merit. In this chapter, we will look at why green tea can be a valuable component of any oral-care plan, especially for preventing cavities, but also with benefits related to gingivitis (gum disease) and bad breath.

Q. How does green tea fight cavities?

A. You may think of cavities as a result of too much sugar. That's only part of the problem. In fact, tooth decay is a result of a complex series of events involving the bacterium *Streptococcus mutans.* This organism, which thrives on sugar, has an affinity for the mouth, where it decays the enamel of teeth, leading to dental cavities. Green tea inhibits the growth of *S. mutans*, as well as other bacterial species associated with dental problems.

Researchers at the Department of Clinical Pathology at Nihon University School of Dentistry in Japan investigated the cavity-preventing ability of green-tea extracts, both in a laboratory setting and in animals. They determined, based on evidence gathered by growing *S. mutans* on saliva-coated discs, that polyphenols from green tea prevented the bacteria from attaching themselves to these simulated teeth. Of all the polyphenols, EGCG was the most powerful cavity-fighter.

Yet another mechanism by which tea polyphenols reduce the risk of cavities is by increasing the resistance of the tooth itself to the actions of cavity-causing bacteria. Researchers from the Department of Preventive Dentistry at Kyushu University in Japan say that tea strengthens the bonds between fluoride and the calcium, phosphorus, and organic substances in tooth enamel, resulting in a tooth surface that is highly resistant to cavity-causing acids produced by bacteria.

Q. Fake teeth in a laboratory are interesting, but what about in real people—can green tea really make a difference?

A. It sure can. In one enlightening study, thirty-five volunteers refrained from brushing, flossing, and all other oral-hygiene procedures for a four-day period while eating a normal diet. Meanwhile, they were given a solution containing tea polyphenols and asked to rinse their mouths with it after each meal and before bed. Before and after the study period, bacteria counts were taken and a dental examination conducted. For a second four-day period, the volunteers repeated the same procedures, but the mouth rinse they were given did not contain any active ingredients.

The results of this study showed that rinsing the mouth with polyphenols greatly reduced plaque deposition, as compared to using the plain mouth rinse. This despite the fact that the volunteers were not brushing or flossing. In thirty-four of the thirty-five volunteers, plaque deposition was clearly decreased, suggesting that the polyphenols have powerful anti-plaque properties.

Q. What about the fluoride content of green tea, which you mentioned in Chapter 1?

A. Many years ago, dental researchers noticed that people living in areas where the drinking water naturally contained fluoride had very few cavities. This led to the movement to add fluoride to drinking water across the country. However, when the fluoride levels are too high, harmless (but unattractive) brown stains can appear on the teeth. Obviously, a balance of fluoride is best for teeth. Experts recommend that 1 part per million (ppm) of fluoride in water is a health-enhancing level. High levels of fluoride (in excess of 8 ppm), can result in the discoloration of teeth, as well as possible bone abnormalities.

Fluoride helps the body to build teeth that are harder, larger, more uniform, and more resistant to decay by acids and demineralization. The benefits of fluoride are greatest when fluoride exposure begins in infancy and continues during tooth development. Experts estimate that as many as half of all cavities could be prevented with optimal fluoride exposure. The fluoridation of municipal water supplies, which began in the 1950s, now covers more than half of the United States population. Many people, regardless of whether their water is fluoridated, also apply fluoride topically during dental visits and via toothpaste.

Green tea is an abundant source of fluoride, which partially accounts for its cavity-fighting properties. Green tea provides fluoride protection in two ways. First, the process of drinking the tea exposes the teeth surfaces to fluoride (in a similar process to anti-plaque mouth rinses or toothpastes). Second, after the green tea is swallowed, the fluoride is absorbed by the body and can be incorporated into the tooth structure.

Q. What about cavities in children?

A. Comparisons of children who drink tea and those who don't suggest that drinking at least one cup of tea daily (as opposed to less than three cups per week) results in a statistically significant improvement in dental health. Other research in school-age children reports that drinking green tea reduces the number of cavities.

Q. What if I already have a cavity?

A. If it's too late for prevention, and a cavity has already developed, green tea might still help. According to traditional healers, the pain of a toothache can sometimes be eased by gently chewing tea leaves or simply pressing the tea leaves against the tooth in question. Meanwhile, of course, you'll want to contact your dentist.

Q. Can green tea do anything else for my teeth?

A. In addition to preventing cavities, green tea can help treat extreme bacteria overgrowth and damage. Polyphenol extracts from four different Japanese green teas were assessed for their antibacterial effects against twenty-four different strains of bacteria found in infected root canals. In devising the study, the researchers theorized that if Japanese green teas could be shown to have an effect on bacteria in infected root canals, then green tea might have some use in treating this condition. True to form, the polyphenols came through as antibacterial agents in this study. The growth of as many as half of the bacterial strains identified were inhibited by the green teas, suggesting that green tea may be a promising treatment for infected root canals.

Q. Can green tea help my gums?

A. Gingivitis, or inflammation of the gums, is a very common condition that is the beginning stage of periodontal disease, which can become quite serious. While gingivitis is reversible, the damage done by periodontal disease is permanent, which is why treatment for gingivitis is absolutely crucial for continued dental health.

The earliest symptom of gingivitis is swollen, soft, red gums that bleed easily. Unfortuantely, this condition often goes unnoticed because it is usually painless. In most cases, gingivitis results from poor dental hygiene practices; proper daily brushing and flossing and regular dental cleanings greatly decrease your chances of developing it. If gingivitis progresses, plaque-filled pockets can form between the teeth and gums. The gums become inflamed, enlarging the pockets and trapping even more plaque. This is periodontal disease. Over time, it can lead to tooth loss.

Gingivitis is often caused by the same bacterial plaque that causes dental cavities, so the same properties that make green tea useful for preventing cavities make it valuable for reducing the risk of gingivitis. Other bacteria that can cause gingivitis are inhibited by green tea also. As with conventional treatment for gum disease, green tea is most effective in the earliest stages, and becomes less effective as gingivitis progresses to the serious condition of periodontal disease.

Q. What about bad breath?

A. Plaque doesn't only cause tooth decay and gum disease. It is also the primary cause of bad breath. The odor of bad breath (or halitosis, as it is known to doctors) comes from a combination of decomposing foods and tissue and bacteria. Although bad breath has been blamed on many foods, including garlic, onions, and cheese, these foods really only serve to make existing bad breath worse. The real cause is plaque. In most cases, if plaque is removed daily (through brushing and flossing) and decayed teeth are cleaned and repaired, bad breath will go away. Rinsing your mouth with green tea, or just swishing a mouthful of green tea around in your mouth, can aid in the prevention and treatment of bad breath by dislodging accumulated food particles, as well as by decreasing the amount of plaque sticking to your teeth.

7.

Making Green Tea a Part of Your Life

By now, you are probably convinced that green tea deserves a place in your life. How can you not be, given the role green tea can play in reducing the risk of heart disease, cancer, and other health problems? But perhaps you're unsure about how to incorporate green tea into your diet. This chapter will answer your questions about how much green tea you should drink, where to find it, how to brew it, and alternatives you can use if you would prefer not to drink green tea every day. If you are concerned about caffeine or side effects from green tea, you will find those issues addressed here as well.

Q. Exactly how much tea do I need to drink if I want to get the benefits you have described in this book?

A. Most of the benefits of green tea were first noted in Asian countries. It therefore makes sense to drink the amount of tea common to those countries. The average green-tea intake in Asian countries is about three cups daily, which translates into a polyphenol intake of roughly 240 to 320 mg a day.

Q. Can I drink *too much* green tea?

A. The long and apparently safe consumption of tea, particularly green tea, by humans confirms that it is safe to use in reasonable doses. Indeed, tea is accepted as a flavoring agent and is listed on the *generally recognized as safe* (GRAS) list maintained by the U.S. Food and Drug Administration (FDA). Studies in animals show that you would need to drink 50 to 100 cups of tea before any toxic reactions developed. It's hard to imagine anyone swallowing that much tea—or any other beverage, for that matter—in one sitting! The most common adverse effect from drinking exceptionally large amounts of tea is the overstimulation and insomnia triggered by caffeine. If you are sensitive to caffeine in this way, you will want to monitor your intake of caffeine from all sources.

Q. Okay, it's safe. But are there any reasons I might not want to use green tea?

A. There really are very few negatives to green tea. The only cautions would be for women who suffer from fibrocystic breast disease or premenstrual syndrome (PMS). They may want to be cautious about their intake of green tea, since some evidence suggests that tea of any kind may actually worsen these conditions. In addition, pregnant women should steer clear of all sources of caffeine, and, if possible, even avoid caffeine for a few weeks before conception takes place.

Q. What is the fibrocystic breast disease connection?

A. At some point in their lives, more than half of all women suffer from symptoms of fibrocystic breast disease. This condition is characterized by painful, lumpy breasts. Its underlying cause is unknown. It is not green tea itself that may affect this condition, but the caffeine it contains. In the early 1980s, one study suggested that caffeine may create an increased risk of developing fibrocystic breast disease. As many as 65 percent of women in this study experienced complete relief from their symptoms when they eliminated coffee, tea, chocolate, and other sources of caffeine from their diets. Subsequent research has not been able to reproduce or confirm this study's results. Nonetheless, some women with fibrocystic breast disease choose to avoid caffeine and report an improvement in their symptoms when they do so. If you feel that your fibrocystic breast disease symptoms are aggravated by caffeine, there is no reason that you cannot drink decaffeinated tea or take caffeine-free green-tea polyphenol supplements.

Q. Does green tea make PMS worse?

A. Premenstrual syndrome (PMS) has been indirectly linked to green tea, and again it is the caffeine that appears to be the culprit. More than 150 different symptoms have been documented in women suffering from PMS, but most PMS sufferers complain of pain, mood changes, weight gain, swelling, breast tenderness, and food cravings, usually starting one to fourteen days prior to the onset of menstruation. Among other dietary changes, some experts recommend avoiding any sources of caffeine to reduce symptoms of PMS.

Dr. Annette MacKay Rossignol of Oregon State University teamed up with Chinese researchers at the Shanghai Medical University to investigate whether green tea influenced PMS. They followed the diets and green-tea drinking habits, as well as the PMS symptoms, of 188 young Chinese women. Tea was the only source of caffeine for these women. The more frequent tea drinkers were found to be more likely to suffer from PMS, particularly if they consumed five or more cups of green tea daily.

Q. What if I don't want to drink green tea?

A. Although the unique aroma and taste of green tea is appreciated around the world, not everyone cares for it. Or perhaps you would rather not drink the multiple cups per day that are associated with disease prevention and treatment. As an alternative, you can buy green-tea extracts in supplement form. Supplemental forms of green tea provide controlled doses of polyphenols so you know exactly how much you are getting. When you brew a cup of tea, polyphenol levels can vary as a result of many factors, including where the tea plant was grown, how it was processed, its age, how you brewed it, and so on. When choosing a green-tea supplement, you will want to look for a standard extract containing up to 97 percent polyphenols (with up to 67 percent being EGCG). The usual recommended dose is 300 to 400 mg daily.

Q. Where can I purchase green tea?

A. Although things are starting to change, green tea is not necessarily something you will find in your local grocery store. Health-food stores are often a better bet. Incidentally, health-food stores are also a good place to find green-tea supplements (your local pharmacy also should carry green-tea supplements). For an extensive green-tea selection, Asian specialty stores are probably the best place to shop.

Q. Are there different kinds of green tea?

A. There are many varieties of tea to choose from,

based on your personal taste. Try several different ones until you find one that suits your taste. Your choices include gunpowder, hyson, dragonwell, matcha, and sencha teas, among others.

Q. Once I have my green tea, do I have to do anything special with it?

A. After you have purchased the variety of tea you desire, it is important to store it correctly. The quality of the tea can easily be degraded if it is stored improperly and allowed to absorb the moisture and flavor of its environment. In addition, tea exposed to the air will lose its flavor as the aromatic oils evaporate. The best strategy is to buy a small quantity of tea at a time and store it in an airtight container in a cool location for no longer than six months.

Q. Are there any special tips for brewing the perfect cup of green tea?

A. Brewing a pot or cup of green tea is a simple process. Basically, you boil water in a kettle and pour it over the tea leaves, either in a teapot or a mug. Of course, the quality of the water is important to the finished product. If your tap water imparts an unpleasant taste to your tea, try using bottled or filtered water instead.

The temperature of the water is also important. Green tea comes out best when the water is brought almost to the point of boiling, but never actually reaches a rolling boil. You might want to swish a little hot water in the teapot to warm it, then empty the pot before combining the water and tea leaves.

Use approximately 1 tsp of leaves for each cup of tea you brew. The leaves should be left in the water for only three minutes (even less for tea bags). Using an infuser or tea ball makes it easy to remove loose tea leaves after brewing the tea; alternatively, you can pour the tea through a fine strainer to remove the tea leaves. Milk, sugar, lemon, and other flavorings are not usually added to green tea–it is simply enjoyed in its unaltered state.

Q. Are there any tricks for reducing the caffeine content of tea?

A. The shorter the brewing time, the less caffeine will end up in the final product. For example, infusing tea leaves in hot water for three minutes results in a cup of tea with a caffeine content of 20 to 40 mg, while just letting the leaves steep for one minute more results in a cup with 40 to 100 mg of caffeine. Also, the size of the leaves affects caffeine levels in brewed tea. A tea bag, which is filled with tiny broken bits of tea leaves, releases twice as much caffeine as the equivalent amount of whole leaves.

Q. By the way, what exactly is the Japanese tea ceremony?

A. The goal of the Japanese tea ceremony is for the host and guests to attain spiritual satisfaction through the drinking of tea and quiet contemplation of the tearoom. The ceremony is a blend of many elements, including the Chinese custom of drinking tea and Zen philosophy. Zen followers believe that enlightenment is attained through meditation, and the tea ceremony is seen as a way to discipline the mind for meditation. In fact, a well-known saying claims that "tea and Zen are one and the same."

Conclusion

Are you convinced yet that you should join in enjoying one of the 1.5 billion cups of tea that the world's tea drinkers enjoy each day? You probably are. When you brew that cup of tea, do yourself a favor and make it green tea.

If you do, you will be getting a powerful dollop of antioxidants and protecting yourself from a wide array of diseases. You will also be boosting your immunity, increasing your feeling of well-being—even warding off the dentist's drill. So whether you drink tea for a morning pick-me-up or enjoy it as part of a soothing ritual in the afternoon or evening (or both!)—you will have found a great way to support your continued good health.

Glossary

Antioxidant. A compound that neutralizes free radicals.

Basal metabolic rate. The rate at which energy is used for maintaining basic body processes, such as breathing and heartbeat.

Caffeine. A natural compound present in tea, coffee, and chocolate. It is a member of a family of chemicals called methylxanthines and acts as a central nervous system stimulant.

Camellia sinensis. Latin name for the tea plant.

Carcinogen. A substance that can cause cancer.

Catechins. Another name for the polyphenols in green tea.

Detoxification. The process of cleansing the body of drugs and other poisons.

ECG. *See* Polyphenols.

EGCG. *See* Polyphenols.

Flavonoids. Substances found in plants that have antioxidant and disease-preventing effects.

Free radical. A highly reactive molecule or fragment of a molecule that can damage cell membranes and other cell components, contributing to degenerative diseases such as heart disease, cancer, premature aging, cataracts, and many other conditions. Free radicals are present in polluted air, tobacco smoke, some foods, pesticides, and ultraviolet radiation. Some also are manufactured during normal body processes.

Oxidation. The process of reacting with oxygen. In the body, oxidation reactions often result in free-radical damage to cells, tissues, and organs.

Polyphenols. Naturally occurring compounds in tea and other plant foods that are powerful antioxidants. The four primary polyphenols in green tea are epicatechin, epicatechin gallate (ECG), epigallo-catechin, and epigallocatechin gallate (EGCG).

Streptococcus mutans. Bacteria in dental plaque responsible for the development of cavities.

References

The information in this book is drawn from several hundred scientific references. Following are some of those references.

Chosa H, Toda M, Okubo S, et al., "Antimicrobial and microbicidal activities of tea and catechins against Mycoplasma," *Kansenshogaku Zasshi (Journal of the Japanese Association for Infectious Disease)* 66 (1992): 606–611.

Elvin-Lewis M and Steelman R, "The anticariogenic effects of tea drinking among Dallas children," *Journal of Dental Research* 65 (1968): 198.

Fujiki H, Yoshizawa S, Horiuchi T, et al., "Anticarcinogenic effects of epigallocatechin gallate," *Preventive Medicine* 21 (1992): 503–509.

Gomes A, Vedasiromoni JR, Das M, et al., "Antihyperglycemic effect of black tea (*Camellia sinensis*) in rat," *Journal of Ethnopharmacology* 45 (3) (1995): 223–226.

Hamilton-Miller JMT, "Antimicrobial properties of tea (*Camellia sinensis* L.)," *Antimicrobial Agents and Chemotherapy* 39 (11) (1995): 2375–2377.

Hayashi M, Yamazoe H, Yamaguchi Y, et al., "Effects of green tea extract on galactosamine-induced hepatic injury in rats," *Nippon Romen Igakkai Zasshi (Japanese Journal of Geriatrics)* 100 (5) (1992): 391–399.

Hirose M, Hoshiya T, Akagi K, et al., "Inhibition of mammary gland carcinogenesis by green tea catechins and other naturally occurring antioxidants in female Sprague-Dawley rats pretreated with 7,12-dimethylbenz[a]anthracene," *Cancer Letters* 83 (1994): 149–156.

Horiba N, Maekawa Y, Ito M, et al., "A pilot study of Japanese green tea as a medicament: Antibacterial and bactericidal effects," *Journal of Endodontics* 17 (3) (1991): 122–124.

Imai K and Nakachi K, "Cross sectional study of effects of drinking green tea on cardiovascular and liver diseases," *British Medical Journal* 310 (1995): 693–696.

Kao PC and P'eng FK, "How to reduce the risk factors of osteoporosis in Asia," *Chinese Medical Journal* 55 (3) (1995): 209–213.

Kono S, Ikeda M, Tokudome S, et al., "A case-control study of gastric cancer and diet in northern Kyushu, Japan," *Japan Journal of Cancer Research* 79 (1988): 1067–1074.

Liao S, Umekita Y, Guo J, et al., "Growth inhibition and regression of human prostate and breast tumors in athymic mice by tea epigallocatechin gallate," *Cancer Research* 96 (1995): 239–243.

Maity S, Vedasiromoni JR, and Ganguly DK, "Anti-ulcer effect of the hot water extract of black tea (*Camellia sinensis*)," *Journal of Ethnopharmacology* 46 (3) (1995): 167–174.

Nakayama M, Suzuki K, Toda M, et al., "Inhibition of the infectivity of influenza virus by tea polyphenols," *Antiviral Research* 21 (1993): 289–299.

Onishi M, Ozaki F, F Yoshino, et al., "Experimental evidence of caries preventive activity of nonfluoride component of tea," *Journal of Dental Health* 31 (1981): 158–161.

Otake S, Makimura M, Kuroki T, et al., "Anticaries effects of polyphenolic compounds from Japanese green tea," *Caries Research* 25 (6) (1991): 438–443.

Rossignol AM, Zhang J, Chen Y, et al., "Tea and premenstrual syndrome in the People's Republic of China," *American Journal of Public Health* 79 (1989): 67–69.

Sadakata S, Fukao A, and Hisamichi S, "Mortality among female practitioners of Chanoyu (Japanese "Tea-ceremony")," *Tohoku Journal of Experimental Medicine* 166 (1992): 475–477.

Sakanaka S, Aizawa M, Kim M, et al., "Inhibitory effects of green tea polyphenols on growth and cellular adherence of an oral bacterium, *Porphyromonas gingivalis*," *Bioscience, Biotechnology, and Biochemistry* 60 (5) (1996): 745–749.

Shim JS, Kang MH, Kim YH, et al., "Chemopreventive effect of green tea (*Camellia sinensis*) among cigarette smokers," *Cancer Epidemiology, Biomarkers, and Prevention* 4 (4) 1995: 387–391.

Stensvold I, Tverdal A, Solvoll K, et al., "Tea consumption. Relationship to cholesterol, blood pressure, and coronary and total mortality," *Preventive Medicine* 21 (1992): 546–553.

Zheng W, Doyle TJ, Kushi LH, et al., "Tea consumption and cancer incidence in a prospective cohort study of postmenopausal women," *American Journal of Epidemiology* 144 (1996): 175–182.

Suggested Readings

Mitscher, Lester A., Ph.D. and Victoria Dolby. *The Green Tea Book: China's Fountain of Youth*. Garden City Park, NY: Avery Publishing Group, 1998.

Antol, Marie Nadine. *Healing Teas*. Garden City Park, NY: Avery Publishing Group, 1996.

Index